Table of Contents

Comprehensive Guide to Managing Lumbar and Hip Arthritis: Medications, Procedures, Therapies, and Home Remedies

1. Introduction to Lumbar and Hip Arthritis

1.1. Understanding Arthritis in the Lumbar and Hip Regions

2. Medications for Lumbar and Hip Arthritis

2.1. Nonsteroidal Anti-Inflammatory Drugs (NSAIDs)

2.2. Analgesics

2.3. Disease-Modifying Antirheumatic Drugs (DMARDs)

Treatment for Arthritis in the Lower Back and Hips

1. Introduction to Arthritis in the Lower Back and Hips

In the United States, more than 12 million people report having arthritis in the hips, and this number is projected to increase to 17 million by 2030. Every year, more than 2 million people visit healthcare professionals in the United States for the treatment of hip pain. According to global figures, the prevalence of hip osteoarthritis in people over the age of 50 ranges from 3.5% to 8.1%, with women being two to three times more likely to develop osteoarthritis than men. According to the Center for Disease Control and Prevention, arthritis, a prevalent illness in the United States, affects 54.4 million adults aged 18 and older. With advances in surgical procedures and technology, significantly more people are now undergoing major lower back or hip surgery. Arthritis that has developed in the lower back or hips can be excruciatingly painful.

Tens of millions of individuals have osteoarthritis, a degenerative joint disease that causes pain and/or stiffness in one or more joints, in the United States. Osteoarthritis of the hips and knees are the most common causes of chronic pain and disability in this community. It is estimated that 15% to 30% of all individuals who suffer from chronic pain are affected by osteoarthritis. While patients with lower back pain frequently develop arthritis in their spine, the chances of developing arthritis in the hips also rise as the illness progresses over time. It is difficult to provide comprehensive treatments for these patients.

2. Understanding the Causes and Symptoms of Arthritis in the Lower Back and Hips

When you have osteoarthritis in the hips, it is common that you will feel pain in the groin and/or down the inside thigh. Pain in the hip and buttock is common, but pain can be referred. It is common that the pain will stop you (often very abruptly), and you will tend to lean away from the painful leg, putting more weight on the unaffected leg. This action is often done quite automatically, so you may not even realize you're doing it. Pain may also be experienced when walking, sitting, or going upstairs. You could need to use your hands to help move your legs as the catching and swelling may restrict the movement in the hip. Lower back symptoms include dull aching pain after activity and may last up to six weeks. Movement can become restricted, and there may be muscle spasms. Pain can also be felt down the thigh, often referred to as sciatica.

Arthritis is a common cause of back pain and disability. It is more likely to progress if you have had a previous back injury or are physically inactive and overweight. Both the lower back and the hips are areas in which arthritis is common. The leading cause of both lower back and hip arthritis is osteoarthritis. Lower back arthritis causes a deep aching pain that is worse in the morning and better in the afternoon. Pain can last up to six months in a single episode and can recur over the years. It is most likely to be triggered by awkward heavy lifting, pushing or pulling, repetitive bending, and twisting as part of one's daily activities.

3. Diagnosis of Arthritis in the Lower Back and Hips

Physical Examination: Movement and Palpation Treatment for arthritis in the lower back and hips is likely to begin with an initial exam, followed by a few tests. During the initial exam, a doctor will ask specific questions about how the pain began. The patient will be asked where it is strongest and if it can be referred. Then, valuable clues may be gathered from watching the patient walk. Although the "duck waddle" gait, or a stiff-legged gait, suggests arthritis is present, the main purpose of watching a patient walk is to determine if there are any signs of a nerve that is being compressed. Blood flow patterns can be helpful in diagnosing sciatica. Typically, obstructed blood flow causes increased pain while walking. When painful walking causes rest, the pain is relieved. It is called intermittent claudication, and it may be an indicator of vascular (circulation) problems. Other gait variations are considered too. When a patient hops on the affected leg to avoid jarring the other leg, this suggests hip disease. When a patient limps in and out of a walking stick, the doctor can deduce from this that there is a spine condition. The patient is then asked to lie flat, and the doctor evaluates how far the knee can be bent and rotated. If range of motion is limited, the problem may be in the hip or spine. If the thigh and leg motions are painful, arthritis is probably a problem. X-rays can help confirm the diagnosis.

Introduction How do doctors diagnose arthritis in the lower back and hips? There are several ways that arthritis can be confirmed. Some of the simple diagnostic procedures are the following: a medical history, physical examination, blood tests, and imaging tests.

3.1. Physical Examination

Physical examination can be broken down into several components. These components are the inspection and documentation of deformities of the extremity, range of motion, muscle strength, palpation of tissues, joint-line tenderness, ligamentous testing, and neurological assessment. The next section will cover each of these aspects of physical examination in detail. It cannot be overemphasized how important physical examination is to good medical care. Experience is important when dealing with physical examination techniques. Practice doing the examination in an orderly fashion. Do it the same way every time, and count on the proper diagnostic maneuver seven to eight out of ten times to give you the answers you need. It is particularly important to have a series of diagnostic tests specific for arthritis in the lower back and hips. These tests, when combined with symptoms and history, allow for an accurate diagnosis of the condition. Only when you can accurately make the diagnosis can you proceed with an appropriate treatment plan.

Physical examination is probably the most important aspect of diagnosing arthritis in the lower back and hips. It is also a critical part of evaluating your treatment. The diagnosis of arthritis is usually made through a combination of taking a history and doing a physical examination. The history typically raises suspicion for arthritis, and the physical examination often helps confirm the diagnosis that is suggested by the history.

3.2. Imaging Tests

Some doctors use ultrasonography (or ultrasound) to look at the ball-and-socket hip joint to help in diagnosing hip arthritis. For a more accurate diagnosis, an ultrasound may be performed by a radiologist, who is a doctor who specializes in medical imaging. Some physicians also use diagnostic, but invasive, imaging techniques for hip arthritis such as arthrography.

Imaging has a limited role in the diagnosis of non-specific lower back pain, since many findings are very common in the general population, but are often unrelated to pain. The following are the relevant imaging tests that can help diagnose arthritis in the lower back and hips: - X-Rays (Radiographs) - Magnetic Resonance Imaging (MRI) - Computed Tomography (CT) - Bone Scan Imaging (Scintigraphy) - Myelography (Myelogram)

Most of the time, arthritis can be diagnosed based on your symptoms and a physical examination. However, the appropriate tests may be ordered to confirm the diagnosis, rule out other causes, or evaluate the extent and location of damage inside the joint. Imaging tests can help diagnose or rule out arthritis in the lower back and hips. These imaging tests can also help your healthcare provider to see the location and extent of arthritis in the spine or hips, as well as any bony outgrowths (e.g. spurs), decreased joint spacing or joint destruction, or loosening of the implant in the case of a joint replacement. Imaging tests can also help to guide some treatments or surgical techniques.

- Magnesium levels and factors to check for any Vitamin deficiencies, such as in Ankylosing Spondylitis.

- Uric Acid and uptake of liver enzymes to check for Gout or any damage to the liver.

- Rheumatoid Factor and Anti-CCP levels to check for rheumatoid arthritis.

- Full blood count to check the general health.

If another major joint is suspected to be affected (e.g. the shoulders or knees), the doctor might request extra blood tests just to make sure that these joints are not affected or assess their severity/cause. Blood tests to indicate severity or causes of arthritis:

- HLA-B27 gene testing, which is most commonly associated with Ankylosing Spondylitis, may be indicated in conjunction with assessment by a specialist. It is more likely in people whose affected family members have Ankylosing Spondylitis or Psoriatic arthritis than those who do not.

- Erythrocyte sedimentation rate (ESR) and C-reactive protein (CRP) are non-specific tests that can detect inflammation in the body. They are not usually related to back pain or hip pain, but they can go up when you are sick. In some cases of arthritis, the ESR and CRP tests can go up. However, many forms of arthritis can be present with normal results. This means if you have a form of arthritis, the tests will not reflect this, but if they do go up at any stage, the consultant may use them to monitor the extent or presence of the disease.

The doctor may request blood tests. These blood tests will not tell you for certain whether or not you have lower back pain or hip pain. They can find out about your treatment. Our options are:

4. Non-Surgical Treatment Options

Lifestyle Lifestyle adjustments can reduce pain by reducing body weight. During walking, the pressure on the areas affected by the arthritis is about three times the body weight. Given that approximately 2-3% less weight helps to reduce pain, loss of 1 kilogram can theoretically reduce body weight by about 3-4 kilograms during walking. Regular exercise, albeit adjusted to individual fitness, stimulates blood flow and metabolism to the rest of the body, including the lower back and hips.

Physical therapy Physical therapy is important for people who suffer from lower back or hip osteoarthritis. It helps improve muscle strength in the legs and abdomen, which reduces the pain caused by the arthritis. It also helps the body to find its balance by working on coordination, which in turn protects the affected joint from overuse.

Medication Pain relief medication, cortisone injections, and local anesthetics all give patients relief from their lower back or hip pain. This allows them to increase their sport and daily activities, allowing them to improve their physical condition crucial for self-management of osteoarthritis of the lower back and hip. Using the temporary relief of pain these treatments offer, patients will be more receptive to physical therapy in order to improve their physical condition.

Non-surgical treatment options for arthritis If you have lower back or hip arthritis symptoms and aren't ready for surgery, or if surgery isn't right for you, it's still possible to find relief. Depending on your specific needs, your doctor can offer you a broad range of non-surgical treatment options to help you manage your symptoms and their progression.

1. Acetaminophen (Tylenol): This painkiller is an analgesic. Its only function is to relieve pain. 2. Opioids: These potent painkillers are used primarily to relieve pain from injury, arthritis, surgery, or cancer. They require a prescription. 3. Nonsteroidal anti-inflammatories (NSAIDs): NSAIDs are painkillers as well as anti-inflammatory drugs for arthritis and related conditions. They limit the body's production of prostaglandins, signaling molecules that cause pain, inflammation, and fever. Acetaminophen, opioids, and NSAIDs only treat the symptoms of arthritis, and they cannot cure the disease itself. However, they can help reduce joint inflammation and alleviate arthritis symptoms. Some NSAIDs are available without a prescription (over-the-counter), while others require a prescription from a doctor. Be sure to check with your doctor before taking an over-the-counter prescription. Remember, safe use of these medications is important, and your doctor will manage them with you.

There are many medications that can help control pain and inflammation. However, among the drugs used to treat arthritis of the lower back and hip are:

Arthritis in the lower back and hips is a common problem. Medications that control pain and inflammation help many people with this condition.

4.2. Physical Therapy

For instance, a patient who is suffering from moderate spinal stenosis of the lower back (and potentially arthritis as well) may get the most relief of pain and discomfort by participating in a physical therapy program. Similar to the cervical spine, the majority of spinal stabilization exercises also help to stabilize and condition the muscles in the lumbar spine. Range of motion exercises enhances the elderly's capacity to perform daily self-care tasks. Results of these gentle exercises appear very promising. All these types of exercises have been shown to be effective for some people who want to manage or reverse lower back pain and eliminate a reliance on most prescription medications.

Physical therapy usually plays a key role in any non-surgical treatment program. The specific physical therapy techniques and exercises the therapist uses will depend on the cause of the patient's sciatica, arthritis, or lumbar stenosis, and the severity of the symptoms. In general, however, the physical therapist tries to increase the patient's active range of motion and reduce pain to enhance mobility and improve overall function. There may also be a focus on correcting poor posture and body mechanics. Back conditioning and strengthening exercises can help to improve the strength, tone, and control of muscle groups for better spinal support. Lower back stress may be relieved by using techniques and exercises to train the muscles of the lower back to stabilize and condition the lumbar spine.

Below are some ways to modify your environment and work processes at home, or any other relevant activities or work to manage physical symptoms. Additionally, we have provided information about aquatic and hydrotherapy, Tai Chi and acupressure, as these have shown to be beneficial to some people managing this condition. During painful dips or when your back is playing up, having an accurate measure of the weight loss as a result of activity avoidance, as additional weight may put strain on your lower back, may help you lose weight you may have missed otherwise. While you may have constipation, you may lose or have a change in bowel habit 2-3 litres of fluid daily in order to prevent constipation, kidney stones, bladder infections and renal and renal disease so as to ensure your body gets enough fluids. If you are involving a doctor or other health care professional, call your doctor or seek immediate help from other services according to the advice in your health cooker after using external ice packs temporary relief to relax tighter upper back muscles affected by arthritis such as the with acupuncture and dry needling and other traditional medicine or energetic approaches 40 minutes from the above cold and warm gel packs. Acupuncture may also prove effective for many people. Do not use heat after arthritic hip surgery and regularly rest, sit and stretch after your treatment. To reduce the strength of the affected muscle, use the other hand to push against 2 or 3 days after a local cortisone inflammation of the hip.

Staying active is important for arthritis management. It keeps joints flexible, which can ease symptoms, and is also good for your general health. Many people are apprehensive about being active if they have arthritis, but generally people with arthritis can exercise without pain getting worse, particularly where they have followed a graded, progressive exercise program (where the amount of exercise or joint use increases slowly to a manageable level). A doctor or physiotherapist can have a role in helping you find out what types of activity are suitable and at what level. A physiotherapist can also be helpful in tailoring an exercise program to your individual level and concerns. In addition to general advice about physical activity, people with arthritis may benefit from specific advice about how to protect the damaged parts of their lower back and one or two "dos and don'ts" related to physical activity and daily living habits. Certain changes may be useful in reducing the effects of the arthritis on a daily basis. This may involve altering your environment, scheduling your activities and/or scheduling breaks to help you manage the effect of the arthritis and your options for relief of symptoms.

5. Surgical Treatment Options

Hip replacement: Total hip replacement or hip arthroplasty is the surgery performed to replace the arthritic hip joint with prostheses to rid the patient of pain and restore function back to the hip joint. There are several ways to perform a hip replacement. They are known as posterior, anterior, anterior-lateral, and lateral approaches. These approaches are based on the surgical path taken to replace the hip joint. Studies have shown all of these approaches can be successful in the correct patient.

Hip: Surgery to directly alleviate pain in the hip joint typically aims to replace the arthritic portions of the hip.

Laminectomy: Laminectomy surgery aims to increase space in the spinal canal by removing the lamina of the affected vertebra. This removes part of the bone and ligament giving rise to compression of nerves in the spine, typically aiding in relieving leg pain and neurologic symptoms.

Spinal fusion: Spinal fusion surgery is aimed at decreasing back pain by preventing movement between one or more vertebral segments. This is attempted by joining two or more adjacent vertebrae to encourage them to grow together and decrease movement or alignment abnormalities at the painful area.

Low Back: Surgery to directly treat the arthritis in the low back typically aims to decrease back pain. These procedures rely on improving stability and alignment of the arthritic areas in the low back, which can include spinal fusion or laminectomy.

When conservative treatments fail, or when pain and function do not improve with non-surgical treatment options, surgical options can be considered. Surgery options depend on the structure in the low back or hip that is causing your symptoms, and include integration of medical history, physical examination, and imaging studies (e.g. x-rays, MRI, CT scan) to tailor a treatment plan to your pain. The following is an overview of surgical options for arthritis in the lower back and hips.

5.1. Spinal Fusion

Spinal fusion has been used for decades to treat segmental motion-induced low back pain of spondylolisthesis, whether of isthmic, degenerative, or post-surgical origin. Spinal fusion is defined as the placement of bone or bone substitute into or through the disc space with the aim of excluding it and preventing further segmental motion. Lateral listhesis often accompanies spondylolisthesis and lumbar spinal stenosis and has been suggested as a lack of stabilizing effect on the affected level. In the last trial on the subject, reduction of the deformity and decompression only were comparable to reduction of the deformity and decompression with additional Phillips instrumentation in overcoming the listhesis and decompressive reduction (in all effects ranging between groups with and without implants).

People with severe arthritis in the lower back and the presence of large osteophytes encroaching or deforming the canal may benefit from a decompression to remove the bony overgrowth. If the adult patient has any lateral listhesis, and especially if it is of more than just a very slight grade, then spondylodesis needs to be performed at the osteophytic levels. It is suggested, rather than definitely recommended, that spondylodesis be performed in an older adult with a spondylolisthesis plus concomitant degenerative spinal stenosis. Parallel to the spondylodesis literature, there are two studies looking at the functional outcome of older adults who had diarthrodial segmental in addition to a decompression compared with those who had a decompression alone. Both studies make suggestions, rather than definite recommendations, and don't help guide clinical practice. The ideal spinal prosthesis is not yet available, so only the fusion option remains for arthritic hips. Spinal fusion, be it of the traditional or the circumferential style, should not be used as a preventative for ladder slippage because there is no objective evidence that is effective for this, and there is a strong correlation with accelerated intervertebral disc disease.

The objective of both a laminectomy and a foraminotomy is to reduce pressure on the affected nerves in the lower back. This procedure can offer considerable relief to people suffering from stenotic changes related to arthritis in the lower back, especially those with symptoms affecting the lower extremities. It is particularly effective for those who are troubled by leg pain. Laminectomy is by no means without potential complications, though surgical outcomes vary considerably. Many patients who have undergone a laminectomy experience significant reduction in low-back pain following surgery.

Laminectomy is another procedure that may be recommended for certain patients with arthritis in the lower back and hips. The laminae are small bones that are part of the spinal column, and they can be surgically removed to relieve pressure on the arteries. The surgical procedure for which the laminae are removed is called a laminectomy. The procedure is often combined with a related surgery known as a foraminotomy. Between the vertebrae, the foramen is a small hole. The spinal cord and its accompanying nerves pass through the foramen in the lower back contained within each vertebra. A procedure called a foraminotomy aims to widen the foramen, thereby relieving the pressure that is put on the arteries that cause weakness and numbness.

5.3. Hip Replacement

This is now far and away the most common hip surgery performed and it is currently being performed at Plateau Partnership Park Surgical Center. As a replacement, or arthroplasty, surgery, sections of a hip are replaced with synthetic implants. The hip joint is a ball and socket joint and the ball, the head of the femur, is typically replaced, and in some cases the socket or acetabulum is replaced as well. In a total hip replacement, typically offered to the very arthritic hip or to young, active patients with end-stage degeneration and/or advanced labral pathology, the entire joint is replaced. In the above surgical scenario, the approach to the hip is the same, the only difference is the extent of the necessary procedures/performed osteotomies. For a patient with primarily arthritic changes (advanced joint space narrowing, osteophytes, some cyst formation) only the ball/head of femur is replaced, in the form of a hemi-arthroplasty, or surface replacement. In simpler terms, surface replacement is a conservative, but still very effective strategy to minimize a patient's risk of ongoing hip degeneration and pain. In an ideal scenario, arthritic changes in the hip are either addressed surgically with a procedure described above or successfully avoided by a more conservative treatment plan. However, the best treatment plan remains quite variable. There are several options for how to best manage, treat, or refer a patient whose pain originates in the hips and I would be pleased to be able to help.

Since my early days of practice, 19 years ago, the recognition of the hip as a pain generator has garnered amazing attention from both health professionals and the public. This seems to be a category of injury/problem area that everyone can identify with. And it has become crystal clear that the range of normal hip mobility encompasses much less range than was once considered normal. Subsequently, perhaps largely due to this, we are seeing hip replacements performed at far younger ages than previously. For several years now, hip replacements have been offered to and have been a very successful long-term solution for degenerative hips, hips with severe arthritic changes, and hips with advanced labral pathology unresponsive to conservative care.

Dr. Roy Gates

6. Alternative and Complementary Therapies

Some people have found relief from acupuncture for arthritis of the lower back and hips. This is a technique where small needles are placed in specific areas of the skin to help relieve pain or reduce the side effects of drugs. Other people have found help from chiropractic care. This is a form of alternative medicine that focuses on the relationship between the body's structure, primarily the spine, and the body's function. They use their hands to help relieve pain in the body. Yet other people have had luck with herbal remedies or nutritional supplements such as glucosamine and chondroitin. Some people have also used a practice called yoga to manage the pain in the lower back. Yoga has been shown to be helpful in relieving chronic back pain. Experts think that by stretching the muscles and relaxing the mind, the brain can help lessen the pain. While it is necessary to take care of your body the best way possible, some of the alternative therapies or treatments can cause damage if mixed with pain medications, so it is important to talk with a doctor about treatments that are underway or being considered.

Alternative and complementary treatments for arthritis of the lower back and hips can be promising. These treatments complement or are used in conjunction with conventional medical care. As with conventional treatments, not all alternative or complementary therapies will work well for everyone. However, they may help decrease the need for medication and may actually help heal or improve the body's function.

6.1. Acupuncture

Acupuncture is derived from traditional medicine and is a popular treatment in Chinese medicine. It usually involves the insertion of solid, sterile needles through the skin and into the body, particularly into areas where nerves, muscles, and connective tissues are stimulated. In the activation, the procedure involves the discharge of neurochemically active substances such as endorphins or enkephalins. People with arthritis seem to respond well to acupuncture. Its analgesic effects are believed to be due, in part, to acupuncture's capacity to stimulate the release of specific pain-relieving chemicals from the brain. A Cochrane review suggested that acupuncture may exert clinical benefits and deserved to be used as a treatment for chronic back pain and hip osteoarthritis.

Acupuncture is a non-conventional therapeutic approach to the management of arthritis in the lower back and hip region. In this section, the principles of acupuncture and the evidence for its potential mechanisms are examined. Arthritis in the lower back and hip is quite common and leads to substantial disability. The intensity of rehabilitation typically provides only a minor relief to this group of patients. As a result, many people turn to complementary medicine. Acupuncture is one non-conventional therapy that is frequently considered an option for individuals seeking relief.

6.2. Chiropractic Care

Several small, randomized controlled trials have investigated the effects of CT on arthritis in the lower back and hips, permitting only limited conclusions about possible benefits of this treatment to be drawn. The potential benefits of CT must be weighed against the risks and costs of this treatment. CT delivers low-dose targeted therapy for people with arthritis in the lower back and hips, and may be helpful in managing some symptoms of these conditions. A full work-up from a chiropractor or other qualified health care individual before treatment begins is always a good idea. People who decide to use complementary health approaches sometimes have negative previous experiences with conventional medical treatments, such as severe side effects. Although complementary health is not necessarily risk-free, it may offer people opportunities for greater involvement in their own health.

Some people who have arthritis in their lower back and hips use an approach called chiropractic. A chiropractor diagnoses, treats, and prevents disorders of the neuromusculoskeletal systems and the effects of these conditions on general health. Some chiropractors also offer other complementary health approaches, also called complementary and alternative medicine. The goal of chiropractic therapy (CT) is to help loosen tight muscles, move stiff joints, and control pain, among other purposes. Currently, researchers are examining several questions about both CT and other complementary health approaches, including whether CT is helpful for people who have arthritis in the lower back and hips.

6.3. Herbal Remedies

The best way to use herbal remedies is under the care of a qualified herbalist, though you can try some of these as teas or cooking herbs. This way, a herbalist can choose the most suitable remedies for your needs, tailor them to your specific needs, and adjust them over time if necessary. While herbal remedies can support other measures in the management of arthritis and function, they are not a cure. Herbal remedies are most effective when used as part of a holistic approach which may include a special diet, hydrotherapy, exercises, and techniques to reduce pain, improve mobility, and release muscle tension. Developing strength, improving balance, and flexibility in a variety of muscles that support the hips and lower back, including quadriceps, hamstrings, and hip flexors, can improve pain.

There are herbs you can use to help manage some of the symptoms and improve function when you have hip or low back arthritis. They may be described as complementary to other treatments. Some of these herbal remedies may be taken orally, either alone or in a blend. With alcoholic extracts (tinctures) and teas, only non-irritant aromatic herbs should be made without oxalated herbs. In addition to taking herbs orally, there may be a benefit of using essential oils in a skin cream or in a bath. Ask a qualified natural and complementary therapist for advice as to which method of application is the most suitable for you. You could be referred to a medical herbalist or an aromatherapist.

7. Pain Management Strategies

7.2 Injection Treatment for Pain: Nonsurgical therapy begins with a simple medical management program, rest, body and chiropractic therapy, covering other recovery from the physiotherapist and physical therapist. It will also make injections in your back made on the following of the lumbar spinal troubles to wear spinal days. You may need to wear problem skin, making it particularly powerful in the front or front of the spine, particularly in the mid-spine made a spinal shot if you have wear reflex or hips. Research shows that the amount of wear and the painful duration of the back can be significantly diminished by such techniques in about 70% of patients. Administering after a steroid and/or numbing injection (long-term) is a blocking method to regulate grief departments.

7. Pain Management Strategies 7.1 Medicines and Surgery: The families and caregivers who make up the team are important members of your pain treatment program. For arthritis, the pain clinic team treats a unique method based on therapy and coping for chronic pain. These treatments could involve various medications and management programs. This will be recommended and linked for you. The first treatments of pain include dietary supplements, rest, exercise, ergonomic and laying techniques, or pain-induced drug therapy. To reduce suffering, for a variety of people, lifestyle changes and medication play a vital part. The first cure, relaxation, medication, and counseling, is

reviewed. You may need to be observed by a pain team including a pain healer, physical therapist, and/or surgeon.

Lower back and hip arthritis may increase pain. Treating pain is highly important for weakening arthritis. It is healthy and helpful to lessen pain. This part will explain the pain management planning and procedure and the different methods for useful pain relief that you can work with.

7.1. Medications for Pain Relief

Other weak opioids that may be used for arthritis in the back and the hip include Tramadol (also known as Ultram and Ryzolt) which has only been studied in the relief of hip arthritis pain. The possibility of a Tramadol use disorder is present, they are prescription drugs. Tramadol, like opioids, should be avoided in patients with illicit substance use and those on opioid use disorder maintenance therapy. There are a few studies that support the use of strong opioids for arthritis pain. There have been two small studies. One study used Oxymorphone; the other used transdermal Fentanyl and found reduced pain and improved function. There have been no studies of strong opioids for arthritis in the lower back. All of the opioids described above can reduce the effectiveness of breathing, appetite, and cause constipation at low doses. Other side effects include sleepiness, nausea, and dizziness. Opioids are likely to stay with a person, creating a high risk of addiction and misuse. Ease of access and increased doses increase a person's risk of overdose leading to death. Lotions are non-prescription drugs.

Analgesics These drugs reduce pain and are usually the first step for treating patients. Acetaminophen (such as Tylenol), either alone or in combination with opioid-like medications such as codeine, is commonly prescribed for people with hip and back joint arthritis. Codeine in various preparations is more prevalent in other countries. It is available by prescription. Most analgesic medications have not been studied extensively for arthritis of the lower back and the use of codeine or other similar products for hip arthritis pain was not well established.

7.2. Injections for Pain Management

These injections can all potentially be repeated because they provide pain relief but do not treat the source of the pain. It is expected that multiple injections may be required over time but will decrease in frequency due to decreased pain and decreased frequency of pain episodes. The amount of relief provided can vary from six hours to four months or more. Some factors, including stress, can potentially decrease the effectiveness of the injections. Another potential side effect of these injections is weakened muscles and discomfort from the shot itself. However, such symptoms are generally mild and short-lived. Injections have relatively low risk if performed by a well-trained specialist in a sterile environment, and outside of allergic reactions, it is uncommon for severe side effects to occur.

Injections for pain management provide targeted relief to areas of the body where pain is isolated. For individuals with arthritis in the low back or hips, injections can provide significant pain relief, which can lead to better function and increased activity. Different types of injections may be used based on the pattern of pain and its source. By far, the most common injections give concentrated treatment at a particular area within the pain path. This includes injections closer to the peripheral nerves, both at the dorsal root ganglion and the periphery, or in close proximity to joints such as the hip joint.

7.3. Nerve Blocks

Healthy nerves, muscles, and spinal joints are entirely encased in connective tissue. As we age and stretch, twist, lift, and wear out our bodies, the inner contents of our spinal joints can bulge through the outer ligamentous coatings. Inside the joints of our spine, the lubricating jelly, called synovial fluid, can leak out and form a cyst, irritating the spinal nerve that runs through the sacroiliac joint and causes arthritic pain. Severe pain is one of the main reasons that doctors use a nerve block for arthritis diagnosis. Chronic pain can be a heavy burden for most people. Nerve blocks are becoming more established as part of arthritis management and also as a means of troubleshooting any problems with the lower back, hips, and even legs. The process of having a nerve block can isolate the source of discomfort and directly target the irritated or damaged nerves. The technique is also minimally invasive, meaning that it is far less disruptive than other operations. Despite the relief it may provide, however, it is not a permanent solution. A nerve block does not cure the problem itself, but the pain relief that can be provided by the injection can give you a chance to return to normal activities.

A nerve block is a targeted injection of medication into or around a nerve. Nerve blocks can be used to assist in diagnosing the causes of new pain or to provide pain relief for arthritis of the lower back, hips, or legs. Nerves are the messengers that carry signals from the source of injury or pain to the brain where the signal is interpreted as pain. By administering a local anesthetic, the functioning of a nerve can be temporarily blocked, which helps to disconnect this pain signal. This short-term block of pain signals can help relieve pain as well as predict whether a more permanent block is likely to provide more long-term pain relief.

8. Nutrition and Diet Recommendations for Arthritis in the Lower Back and Hips

What is in My Grocery List? Dairy: Extremely low in fat, no fat and low in cholesterol, cereals and breads that are whole grain. Balance these with little amounts of low carbon vegetables and sugar, very few pastas and an intake of rice. For example, eat a $3 box of rice instead of spending $3 and eating cup and 1/4 of packaged rice. Only between 50 to 60 grams of rice will be added to recipes like soups and stews. Fish and Meats: Less fat fish that are rich in omega-3 fatty acids, lean meat, skinless poultry, whole cuts of meat (not the process lunch meats or hot dogs), ground turkey breast instead of whole turkey. If the budget does not allow regular purchase of lean meats and/or fish, eat lesser amounts of meatless meals. Fats and Oils: Liquid oil such as olive oil, canola oil, peanut oil, and low-fat margarine as your primary fat. At a maximum of 6 teaspoons or one serving each day, choose a low fat, trans fat-free mayonnaise and use a small amount of low fat masterpiece on your bread. Use others, like canola or sesame seed for a marinade or dressings since their flavors are more robust. Fruits and Vegetables: For their fiber, nutritional, and calcium-adding values, the amount of calcium in sodium, eat three or more 3-cup servings of green leafy vegetables and include fruits high in vitamin C. Two more colors of fruit or high-fiber juices must be purchased for the nutritional value and potential. Low-fat Foods: Whole grains, bread and flour, trying only small amounts at one time due to the high fat content. 1 tablespoon once a week, like organic peanut butter, if the budget allows. Put one-percent low fat as skim milk, baby as 1% cheese, organic skim milk, or whole dairy products in.

This approach has been around for centuries and found to have some success in managing inflammatory diseases. Taking both an alternative medicine and a traditional medical approach to manage arthritis has been found to be a more effective combination than taking either by itself.

To maximize good nutritional choices, eat a diet high in vegetables, fiber, complex carbohydrates, and in combination with lean meats for the protein needs in our diet, 'good' fats low in cholesterol. Choose from the wide variety of fruits and vegetables that are available and if it is possible select from those that are organically grown or free of chemicals. It might be helpful for some people to limit how much oily fish they eat, such as tuna, salmon, herring, and mackerel because some people will develop fish oil allergies. It is not known if any weight loss could help some people with arthritis. What is known is that losing 10 pounds can take up to 40 pounds of pressure off the weight-bearing joints in the legs and can promote less pain in weight-bearing related joints. A registered dietitian can help identify therapeutic diets to aid in many ways to manage the pain and symptoms of inflammatory diseases. Simply put, therapeutic diets are ones that have been shown to aid in managing a specific disease state.

Chronic diseases cause conditions that include better nutrition and more of it that might otherwise follow. When something that is eaten is causing inflammation, it is likely that pain and quality of life may become worse. Reducing inflammation in the body by eating a healthy diet can be a first step to managing arthritis. Follow these recommendations from the Alternative Medicine Center at A.G. Holley Hospital to help manage arthritic conditions affecting the lower back and hips:

9. Prevention and Lifestyle Tips to Manage Arthritis in the Lower Back and Hips

Lifestyle management: If you have been diagnosed with arthritis in the lower back or hips, try the following lifestyle management techniques: - Occupations that are less physically demanding might reduce the risk of arthritis in the lower back and hips. - If you are overweight, losing weight – especially around the hips and stomach – will reduce the pressure on the lower back and the hips. Weight loss is especially important for those with osteoarthritis in the hips. Once arthritis forms, body weight has the most impact on hip arthritis because the hips carry the brunt of excess weight. - Wear flat, comfortable shoes with good support. - Use cushioned insoles to reduce stress on the lower back and hips. - Using a footrest or stool can also take some stress off the lower back and hips. With your knees lower than your hips, hip joint stress is reduced. - Take a proactive role in managing your diabetes, hypertension, and high cholesterol, as these are risk factors for progressive arthritis of the lower back. - Limit toxic habits, including alcohol, and stop smoking for prevention and overall health.

Prevention tips: Here are some ways you can help prevent arthritis from developing in the lower back and hips: - Exercise: Regular movement may help reduce inflammation in the body. - Wear the right shoes: Keep your body supported and reduce the risk of falling by wearing supportive, protective footwear. - Lift properly: When lifting heavy items and boxes, remember to lift from the legs rather than the back to prevent injury.

Preventing arthritis in the lower back and hips isn't always possible, but there are things you can do to reduce the effect it has on your life. If you do have arthritis, the following management techniques may help you live a healthier, more comfortable life.

Comprehensive Guide to Managing Lumbar and Hip Arthritis: Medications, Procedures, Therapies, and Home Remedies

1. Introduction to Lumbar and Hip Arthritis

The major purpose of using treatment for lumbar and hip pain is to reduce pain and increase function. After the lumbar and hip pain treatment, the goal is increased dynamically. Lumbar and hip surgeries are quite successful in terms of achieving 100% full function in the coming years. The surgeries consist mainly of decompression, eliminating pain, and reducing the severity of other symptoms. However, fractures, dislocation, nerve damage, disc, and other disorders are treated before undergoing the surgery. The common causes for the lumbar and hip joint are fractures of the pelvis, changes in clot, antiphospholipid syndrome, ankylosing spondylitis, benign tumor, abnormal changes in the spine, as stated in Chiari malformation.

The comprehensive guide aims to provide accurate and effective medications, procedures, therapies, and home remedies to manage lumbar and hip arthritis. Lumbar and hip arthritis are quite common, and many people suffer from arthritis globally. Do you know what your body system manages when we sit, walk, and jump? It is your hip. And the next system that joins the hip is the lower back. When the hip gets injured or the lumbar gets injured, it affects the other and makes the situation worse than a single injury. If the hip and lumbar are the main parts in the body, can you ignore their pain? The pain from the lumbar and hip can make the runner, athlete, professional,

and every person inactive. So it is necessary to undergo
lumbar and hip pain treatment.

1.1. Understanding Arthritis in the Lumbar and Hip Regions

The hip is a common source of arthritis due to athletes developing femoroacetabular impingement (FAI), decreased joint space, and increased stress resulting in labral tears and cartilage damage. All these factors contribute to the rise of total hip replacement. Patients suffering from arthritis of the hip undergo decreased hip range of motion, gait disorders, and lateralization of the trunk. As in the lumbar spine, hip arthritis is linked to neurological, metabolic, functional, emotional, and social deprivation. Rates of living with pesky joint arthritis into old age have increased. Pain and changes in activities of daily living are the resulting onset. Auxiliaries in rejuvenating and managing arthritis of the spine and hips include medications, procedures, conventional physical therapy, alternative therapies, and manipulation/hands-on therapy.

The prevalence of lumbar and hip arthritis has seen a rise in an aging population dealing with degenerative wear and tear of the spine and hip joints, as well as in the younger athletic population. The dislocation of the thoracic and lumbar segments in the spine has inevitable degenerative changes due to the aging process. A misaligned spine leads to excess stress in the higher stress point and exacerbates symptoms. Arthritis in the lumbar region can result in back pain, reduced range of motion, and lateral recess stenosis. Due to degenerative changes, root pain often coexists with leg pain in these patients. Lumbar arthritis and stenosis are accompanied by neurological, functional, social, emotional, and economic deprivation.

2. Medications for Lumbar and Hip Arthritis

There are many different classes of medications used to manage arthritis. Although every class of medication has been studied for arthritis of the lumbar spine, not all medications have been studied for arthritis of the hip. Although there is more evidence for treatments of the lower back, we have noted when there is little to no evidence for treatments of the hip. There are two main reasons to use medications for knee and hip arthritis: 1) To manage the symptoms of knee and hip arthritis. Medications used do not change the progression of arthritis but can help with pain, stiffness, and function. 2) To try and slow down the progression of knee and hip arthritis to avoid or delay surgery. Some medications can have a protective effect on the joints, slowing down the wear and tear of arthritis or can help to rebuild components of the joint, like cartilage, that are breaking down. Many medications have been studied for arthritis, including medications that can be found over-the-counter (without a prescription) and medications that require that patients have a prescription from their doctor to use.

The arthritis guide aims to help individuals with arthritis of the lower back and hip understand their medications, procedures, therapies, and home remedies. We explain medication options in detail since many over-the-counter (OTC) and prescription medications are being used. Our goal is not only to help understand these medicines, but also how they may or may not help and appropriate uses for different kinds of medications. Managing arthritis has two key components: treating symptoms and slowing the progression of arthritis. If you have arthritis of the lumbar and hip, this section will help you understand the many different kinds of medications used to treat arthritis.

2.1. Nonsteroidal Anti-Inflammatory Drugs (NSAIDs)

Long-acting NSAIDs are available as topicals and orals. Orals have various release forms, including tablets that gradually release in the body over time or special capsule forms that provide morning and evening release. Diclofenac is an oral NSAID you can buy over the counter as a topical. The American Academy of Orthopedic Surgeons conditionally recommends (suggests) diclofenac capsule to be preferred in primary care because of the more predictable and less variable blood levels it gives in comparison with tablets. Other long-term NSAIDs include etodolac, diflunisal, flurbiprofen, nabumetone, and salsalate. Some of these long-term NSAIDs, such as nabumetone and salsalate, have other drugs attached to them. For example, nabumetone is made up of two chemicals that differ from the parent drug and may result in decreased side effects.

Nonsteroidal anti-inflammatory drugs (NSAIDs) are commonly used for arthritis symptoms. They are considered as tools for managing mild symptoms and, if well managed with a physician, may be used long-term. NSAIDs help manage pain and improve function by blocking one of the enzymes that produce chemicals called prostaglandins. Prostaglandins are involved in the production of inflammation. At a time when inflammation is doing more harm than good, like in arthritis, blocking the production of prostaglandins better manages symptoms of arthritis.

Nonsteroidal anti-inflammatory drugs (NSAIDs) Many medications, procedures, and therapies can be used as potential options for the management of lumbar and hip arthritis. Whether you are considering your first options, or your pain symptoms have changed and it is time to explore new possibilities, consult your physician to identify an approach that will meet your needs and goals. Would you like to speak with someone about this treatment right now?

2.2. Analgesics

Analgesics or pain relievers are an essential part of treating osteoarthritis and can help maintain a good quality of life along with an exercise program and physical therapy. Analgesics can alleviate pain in all areas of your body. Paracetamol (acetaminophen) is the first-line pain medicine for all patients with pain from osteoarthritis. Each patient should consult their healthcare provider to explore their options. It is also important that research has shown that anti-inflammatory medication, or drugs that minimize inflammation, are not as effective in treating chronic pain as previously thought. In an update to its 2018 guidance, the American College of Rheumatology and the Arthritis Foundation strongly recommended topical NSAIDs over oral NSAIDs for knee, hip, and hand osteoarthritis. It is also important that there are limits when it comes to using analgesics. It is possible to become dependent on narcotic pain relievers. If the use of this pain reliever is indicated, a healthcare provider should be consulted. Furthermore, such painkillers raise the risk of death in individuals who use them inappropriately.

Pain-relieving medications constitute the core of lumbar and hip osteoarthritis management. Analgesics are ranked based on their pain-relieving effects. Paracetamol sits atop the pyramid and is the first-line treatment for every osteoarthritis patient. Nonsteroidal anti-inflammatory drugs (NSAIDs) are often prescribed by the surgeons as the next line of therapy per the British Society for Rheumatology guidelines. Opiates are less effective than

NSAIDs but may be taken into account. Antidepressants and antineuropathic agents can be used adjunctively for moderate and severe pain.

2.3. Disease-Modifying Antirheumatic Drugs (DMARDs)

Since all interventions are designed to give symptomatic relief, DMARDs (disease-modifying antirheumatic drugs) for immune-mediated non-infectious arthritis of the peripheral joints are not recommended, particularly for spinal arthritis, including lumbar and hip joint arthritis. If complete pain relief without the need for over-the-counter (OTC) analgesics or physical intervention (procedure or therapy) is your primary goal, concepts related to DMARDs can be for educational purposes only. DMARDs could potentially be helpful to, in theory, address the root pathophysiologic mechanism responsible for causing your specific type of suffering. DMARDs may be prescribed either as monotherapy or in conjunction with another DMARD without significantly compounding side effects. A few DMARD-associated side effects, though rare, are fatal (part of the reason a prescriber may require a mandatory period of being "on-treatment" prior to making a switch or augment). Typically, it takes several weeks to a few months to determine if you are responding to a new DMARD, as well as if your side effects are manageable. Unlike NSAIDs (i.e. Meloxicam), which provide an immediate reduction in pain, DMARDs may be titrated to an effective dose slowly over a period of several weeks to a few months. DMARDs have been demonstrated to postpone joint destruction as part of longitudinal research of individuals with rheumatoid and psoriatic arthritis. Be sure to consult with a rheumatologist or another individual or your specialist about taking DMARDs to address any questions or to confirm the relevance of any elements of this portion of Lumbar Arthritis DDx to your clinical practice.

2.3. Disease-Modifying Antirheumatic Drugs (DMARDs)

2.4. Corticosteroids

Corticosteroids can provide arthritis pain relief, both as a tablet and as a local injection. The reduction of inflammation and other effects can also slow down joint damage. For arthritis in the lumbar spine, corticosteroid injections can appear quite effective for localized back pain and nerve pain. The combination of corticosteroid injection and exercise (physiotherapy) seems to be so effective that this option can be used as a way to avoid using opioids. They are rarely used for people with osteoarthritis in the lower back where nerves are not affected. These can be particularly useful if symptoms are severe and treatment hasn't worked yet and disc damage or nerve pain has occurred. These are stronger anti-inflammatory medicines than NSAIDs, but your doctor will want to limit the number of these tablets you take because of their many side effects. Also, your doctor may not want to continue slimming on a regular basis if taking steroid tablets regularly because of the risk of side effects like heart problems (hypertension or heart failure) and stomach ulcers.

Corticosteroid medications can be given orally (by mouth), injected into a joint or the soft tissue surrounding a joint, or sprayed into the nose. These drugs reduce inflammation throughout the body. They slow the immune response, which lowers the risk for joint damage. Shots given directly into the affected joint or the surrounding tissue can result in temporary pain relief, lasting a few days to a few months. A few studies taking shots of corticosteroids into the facets of the spine or the sacroiliac joint showed some potential effectiveness in increasing pain function, especially at the hip but not lasting 12 weeks. The evidence for benefits of steroids into the greater trochanter for hip arthritis is unknown.

3. Procedures for Lumbar and Hip Arthritis

There are several techniques for managing lumbar and hip arthritis. These techniques focus on provocative techniques to identify candidates that contribute to pain generation, as well as indication confirmation techniques that focus on addressing structural and physiological causes of inflammatory arthritis. People who are considering new interventions for management need clarification on allergic therapies, but the symptoms it generates in the skin and tissues of the body can be addressed from the lens of everyone's opinion.

Managing arthritis of both the lumbar and hip can be done with different treatments. Medication therapy is available for both conditions. It is important to understand the risks and benefits, along with follow-up interventions if medication intervention alone is not effective. In the joint and hip, lateral arthritis, exercise and physiotherapy can help prevent pain medication and situations that require quantifying lateral hip pain and necessary palliative approaches. The same is true for managing both spinal osteoarthritis pain. Evidence shows that upright loading mechanisms in the technique can reduce cartilage and reductions in cartilage are associated with poorer diagnoses, not only in terms of time but also in terms of quality.

For lumbar and hip arthritis, medication therapy and physiotherapy can prevent the need for excessive exercise and reduce pain. There are many different approaches that exist to manage the symptoms and underlying issues caused by arthritis of the lumbar spine and hip.

3.1. Injections (Corticosteroids, Hyaluronic Acid)

In case you have morphological changes at the level of the affected hip, knee, or any other limb, apart from reducing the intensity of the pain, the main objective is to prevent the progression of these morphological alterations of the joints. Therefore, No Excuse can support your recovery by implementing specific physiotherapy programs, and by pursuing a suitable diet program. Our main target is to physically stabilize and protect these joints (mostly by favoring the functioning synergy of the neurotransmitter system) by maintaining a good muscular balance to reduce the pressure and shrinkage of the facet joints. Moreover, the effectiveness of corticosteroid injections is a very good indicator related to the pain source (in the same way as diagnostic injections), which over 50% of the patients get referred to from the knee to other joints. Furthermore, if there has been a positive development, there will be a reduction of the edema back to the normal one that is around one week from the corticoid application. Therefore, the injection can exacerbate the swelling; however, this may also result in reduced pain. Knowing that mosaicplasty in most cases works effectively, some people are desirous to undergo this kind of treatment rather than rehab. The full details on ginex plasty will be in the following tips.

Two of the most common types of injections are corticosteroids (steroids) and hyaluronic acid (viscosupplementation). The main purpose of steroid injections is to alleviate inflammation and give you better pain relief, while visco injections are mainly to provide a "shock absorber" and thus reduce the amount of pain. Both types of injections are primarily aimed at reducing the pain at the level of the affected joint and the radiating ("referred") pain. This pain relief does not last in all patients. For some patients, an ultrasonographic injection technique is chosen, for other patients an X-ray examination (fluoroscopy) is preferred as an injection technique. Both types of injections are performed under local anesthesia that will be discussed on the day of the visit. It is medically justified not to administer any medication prior to the corticosteroid injection procedure since the corticosteroids will be applied directly into the relevant region. Keep in mind that the obvious reason for an injection is to provide pain relief that results in a better quality of life. These injections will keep reducing the pain only as long as the cephalgia you experience is directly related to the arthritis. On the other hand, if you have mainly neuropathic pain, the pain relief you get will last only for head that is not affected either by lameness or a non-physiological movement pattern (viscogenic pain).

Injections

3.2. Radiofrequency Ablation

During the procedure of radiofrequency ablation, a narcotic will be used to sedate the patient, with additional local anesthesia used if the clinical findings and history suggest it is appropriate. The doctor will monitor the patient's heart rate, blood pressure, and oxygen level if the procedure occurs in an outpatient center or hospital setting. A catheter is addressed on the skin and the radiofrequency waves are generated, resulting in heat being emitted, for reasons outlined below. Keep in mind that the path the clinician decides to take during the procedure will be based exclusively on anatomic issues, such as the presence of hardware along the spine, and other clinical factors.

Radiofrequency ablation is focused on specifically addressing the pain caused by arthritis because the sensory nerve of the facet joint, lumbar discs, and sacroiliac joints may become inflamed along with arthritis. The aspect of a nerve that affects sensation can begin to generate pain as well, and these plainly speaking 'pain' signals can travel to the brain. In the past, fusion surgery used to be the only option to decrease pain originating from an arthritic joint. But the minimally invasive procedure of radiofrequency ablation has increased in popularity. The following is a discussion of the principles behind radiofrequency ablation and the specifics of how it is performed.

3.3. Joint Replacement Surgery

Joint replacement requires a prolonged and steady commitment to physical therapy and exercise. It is also important to be aware that the lifespan of joint prostheses is limited. The amount of time a prosthesis will last will depend on the patient's physical activity level, age, and other individual characteristics that make the patient unique. This decrease in the mechanical strength of the prosthesis due to aging or wear may require future revision surgeries to replace the joint prosthesis with new ones. This is usually a bigger concern for younger individuals who undergo joint replacement as the length of time a prosthesis will last is significantly reduced if the patient is young. For this reason, patients may be advised to wait to undergo the procedure, if possible (however, this decision should be individually discussed with the surgeon to review the risks and benefits).

Joint replacement surgery: In many cases, once arthritic pain and nerve compression start to significantly affect one's life, a definitive intervention is required. Joint replacement surgery, also known as total joint arthroplasty, is a proven and extremely effective treatment for advanced arthritis of the lumbar spine and hip joint. It is important to note that in the vast majority of cases, a trial of conservative treatments (usually lasting 6 to 12 months) will generally be recommended before considering this type of surgery. For individuals with end-stage spinal arthritis, joint replacement can result in lasting pain relief and improved function. In general, overall success rates are as high as 90% at 10 years after surgery (for both the hip and for certain types of lumbar spine arthritic conditions).

4. Therapies for Lumbar and Hip Arthritis

The treatment of lumbar and hip OA has evolved from palliative care to procedures that help regenerate joint harm. However, more research is needed to determine the efficacy of new therapies. It is currently recommended that therapeutic advantage be considered on the foundation of the things described above: the signs, impacts of medications, imaging findings, healing coaching, personal preference, and so on.

Considering these holistic methods will enlighten our patients about the variety of ways available for arthritis pain management. There are numerous alternatives to select from as well. Many patients become discouraged when medications are insufficient. If our patients are aware of the entire range of therapeutic choices, they will be able to work with their clinicians to put together a tailored care plan that suits their specific set of circumstances and objectives.

Mind-body approaches: To lessen anxiety and distress. Learn about how to protect the remains of your body. Increase your understanding of how to shift and rearrange activities and purposes during your everyday life.

Manual Therapy: Focuses on providing relief. Train your muscles and bones. It works with your spine to improve actions.

Exercise: As indicated, physical activity may help to lessen discomfort and maintain weight, improving the chance that you can decrease the stress on your bone structures.

When it comes to cases of arthritis, especially in the lumbar and hip areas, painkillers alone can't provide full relief. Many non-pharmacological therapies help manage your arthritis besides pain medication, which many clinicians have said can help alleviate arthritis symptoms. If you want to regain function of your lumbar and hip and improve the quality of your life despite your lumbar and hip arthritis, consider the following therapeutic concepts:

Section title: Therapies for Lumbar and Hip Arthritis

4.1. Physical Therapy

Considerations: While the following benefits of therapy are important, the patient should move and perform those exercises or activities that are biomechanically sound and pain-free. Following the LACC or LACLDs diagnosis, the "no pain, no damage" principle applies, and the therapist will work with the patient to determine safety of exercises or activities. There are many therapeutic claims and many products or "cures" of arthritis.

Benefits and Potential Possible Expected Outcomes: - Establish an exercise program, which is now broken down into the: 1) acquisition phase; 2) consolidation phase; and, 3) maintenance phase - Initial "acquisition phase" focuses on active movement and flexibility exercises to reduce stiffness and improve flexibility - As flexibility improves through the "consolidation phase," correcting muscle imbalance and strengthening to eliminate pain generators takes place

Objective and Purpose: As a therapeutic modality, physical therapy can help patients with arthritis of the low back and hips in many ways. Therapy can address pain, strength, flexibility, range of motion, gait (how patients walk), balance, and function. Once a proper diagnosis is made, it is important to set up a specific end goal - both for the patient and therapist. For example, a patient's end goal may be "I would like to garden again," to which a therapist may suggest walking, balance activities, core strengthening, hip range of motion, and flexibility exercises, which all can be done in the therapy clinic. From here, the patient and therapist can then set marks or short-term goals to finally reach that "end goal." However, if the end goal is unrealistic or not feasible in the short- or long-term, then we will need to revisit the diagnosis, objective testing, and long-term patient goals.

4.2. Occupational Therapy

Some offsets that may have led you to consider skipping occupational therapy may include not feeling prepared to make environmental changes, scared of how "different" it feels to do a specific task "out of the ordinary," or concerns about identifying with a condition based on how you perform tasks. The goal of occupational therapy, however, should not be to make drastic changes at all, but to do what feels comfortable and gets you a bit of independence, freedom, or overall improvement.

Occupational therapy is not a "cure" for arthritis or a way to "get back to normal" quickly. It is a way to learn about how you might improve your daily performance and enable yourself to have a better quality of life. These specialists understand varying degrees of strength, daily function, cognition, and numerous other variables. They are likely encouraging, and sometimes can be a place for you to get the comprehensive assessment needed for a further evaluation. This might be the next step if physical therapy alone does not bring about some boosts in your day-to-day performance. These therapists are typically more accustomed to working with adaptive equipment as well. Offsets of Occupational Therapy

Occupational therapy is a form of therapy that can help you work through your day-to-day life with arthritis. Unlike physical therapy, occupational therapy addresses mainly the functional aspects of the day, which may include dressing, undressing, rolling over, transferring out of bed or off the couch, and getting in and out of a car. You may learn how to perform modified skills, adjust your environment to fit your abilities, use helpful gadgets, or become more accustomed to your current or new equipment. An occupational therapist works in conjunction with a physical therapist and sometimes with a speech therapist to understand how to adjust your life or make the world around you more accommodating. While physical therapy will focus on ways to improve performance and manage an illness through a more active approach, an occupational therapist will often concentrate on how to continue functioning when a full return to day-to-day activities could be unrealistic, for example, to obtain some freedom in the face of a disease or issue that causes extreme disability.

4.3. Aquatic Therapy

The decision to participate in pool classes or use hydrotherapy as a management tool for lumbar and hip conditions and arthritis can be a daunting one. Clinicians at Bodyatwork believe your decision to access our hydrotherapy pool and care in this format may be influenced by discomfort associated with exercising in water, potential risks of exacerbating current symptoms or creating new ones, fears or concerns about how other people will view you in such an environment, and difficulties associated with transferring into the pool and using the pool facilities.

In an aquatic therapy session, a range of factors will be considered. These include the temperature of the water (which is usually warmer than a plunge pool), the depth of the water (to determine load on joints), the intensity of exercise, patient balance, and water buoyancy. The aim of aquatic therapy is to reduce the impact of arthritis for walking, stair management, general activities, and sleeping by improving hip and lumbar movement and mobility. Outcomes can be visible in reduced stiffness after exercise and improvements in activities.

The benefits of the aquatic environment are numerous. Water provides a unique multi-dimensional level of resistance due to its buoyancy factor. Or, in simple terms, joints and muscles can be unloaded, reducing the additional pressure through the lumbar spine and hips during weight-bearing activities.

5. Home Remedies and Lifestyle Changes

Medications, procedures, and therapies for arthritis can be complemented by the following home remedies and lifestyle modifications. Strengthen the muscles in your back and abdomen. Mix up your exercise routines. Exercise at a low level of diversity and in order to acquire a new motion. Regular stretching. Maintain a perfect weight. Use proper lifting techniques. Quit smoking. Posture care. Manage stress. Get adequate sleep and proper rest (7-9 hours). If these suggestions, along with our level one treatments, are insufficient in treating your arthritis, Level Two Treatment may be the best option for you. For instance: regenerative medicine, advanced biologics, stem cell therapy, and alternative pain management.

Home remedies for arthritis (in general) are frequently offered. Given the relatively benign nature of these recommendations, I don't personally have any objection to them, but neither do I believe that they stand to make a great deal of difference, mainly because the problem of osteoarthritis (or degenerative disc disease) occurs internally. Although lifestyle changes may not directly affect the nature or degree of arthritic change, they can significantly affect the comfort and function of an arthritic joint. Joint pain is a significant source of production loss in the economy, and arthritis is among the most costly musculoskeletal disorders.

5.1. Exercise and Stretching

Exercises should be simple, quick, easy, and require no extra equipment. Exercises should be performed on a comfortable and firm surface, such as a carpet or yoga mat, and should be started in the morning and repeated in the evening to improve overall joint health. All exercises should be performed 10 times each and held for 5 seconds. If lying on the back causes severe pain in the knee or lumbar spine, place a pillow under the foot in the supine exercises to slightly bend the knee, relieving tension off the low back. The overall goal of stretching the hip flexors is to have the equivalent flexibility of placing your body flush against a wall while maintaining a posterior pelvic tilt. If a patient can't perform the hip flexor stretch with the primary technique, an alternative version is lying on one side with the bottom leg straight and the top knee flexed on an exercise ball, which raises the top knee and opens the hip on that side, stretching the hip flexor.

Exercise and stretching are essential interventions for patients who have arthritis in their lumbar spine, sacroiliac joints, and hip joints. Exercise increases the secretion of chemicals in the body that are natural pain relievers, such as beta-endorphins. It also strengthens the musculature around the painful joints so that the joints move more efficiently and with less pain. The most effective exercise regimen involves flexibility (stretching) and conditioning (strengthening) exercises, as well as the improvement of cardiovascular health. As with any other exercise program, patients should first be cleared by their primary care physician to participate. Less than 10% of the time, beginning an exercise routine will worsen a patient's symptoms. The majority of the time, a patient will experience an improvement in symptoms.

5.2. Hot and Cold Therapy

One way of managing lumbar and hip arthritis is to modulate the body temperature localized at the site of osteoarthritis. One classic way to directly modulate temperature is through hot and cold therapy. The effects of these therapies were reviewed in the US White Paper titled "Non-Pharmacologic Therapies for Osteoarthritis," and a review of therapeutic modalities found 61 randomized trials spanning January 2006 until June 2011. It was found that heat warmed tissue within 2-3 cm of the skin surface, effectively reduced localized pain, improved general pain, function, and ability not to lose weight. Deep heat was created using fluidotherapy, ultrasound, and lasers. Local warming could provide a considerable analgesic effect and reduce the thickness of subchondral bone. The mechanisms of heat energy are not completely understood and may include increasing the tissue temperature on and within the skin, increasing circulation, decreasing muscle spasm, inhibiting H-reflex with direct effects on muscle contractile stimulators, and metabolic effects such as increased collagen elasticity, relaxation of muscle tone, and relatively decreased motor nerve conduction time.

Hundreds of body temperature-focused products are available for direct use in the form of packs at varying temperatures. These approaches include natural hot springs, more than 15 hydrotherapy pools with a thermal treatment between 36°C (97°F) and 42°C (108°F), mud spas, and thermal mineral-induced springs immersion and showers with a temperature between 36°C and 50°C (97-

122°F). Additionally, a traditional Japanese form of bathing called balneotherapy is performed in Japan to prevent work-related musculoskeletal health impacts, and this involves soaking in water at 41.0°C for 30 minutes three to five times per week.

5.3. Diet and Nutrition

Here's some advice on what to eat to help manage your arthritis in the lumbar and hip areas. Eating a snack that aids in joint lubrication gives lumbar arthritis patients the strength to keep going. Omega-3 fatty acids and their anti-inflammatory properties are supposed to help manage arthritis. Consider moderate consumption of oily fish such as salmon and mackerel, flax, and hemp. Germany's Society for Nutrition, on the other hand, states that a benefit from the intake of isolated omega-3 fatty acids by patients with established arthritis has so far appeared unproven. Since then, study results have not been available. In India, for example, the spice turmeric used in curries has been used for generations to combat arthritis. Its yellow dye has an anti-inflammatory action. Ground turmeric can be added to many dishes as needed.

Tea and curry are only two of the possible ways you can use your diet and nutrition to help manage your arthritis. Here's a quick look at what's happening in managing arthritis in your lumbar and hip regions with diet and nutrition. The connection between diet and arthritis has received a lot of attention recently. The Mediterranean diet, in particular, has been linked to a lower risk of developing arthritis. While the mechanisms remain unclear, some believe that anti-inflammatory fatty acids, vitamins, and minerals in the diet could have something to do with it.

5.4. Ergonomic Modifications

- Raise the chair to the individual's preferred height by using a seat cushion. There is also better uptake of posture and core muscles when people look down at computer monitors and other people from this angle. The pad's material should not cause stress; rather, it should be made of soft, supportive material that can be molded to the individual's shape. The pad's texture should also be smooth, allowing for a sliding motion. The chair should be cushioned or made using a soft material. A forward-leaning, stacking church chair or a folding lounge chair positioned up against a wall to hold it in place are other options. Ergonomic environments for those with lumbar and hip arthritis should be relaxed and easily modifiable in order to optimize comfort. Ergonomic counseling provides resources for professionals; see references and resources: Eastell.

- An adjustable chair can be beneficial. On days when muscles are exceptionally sore, one can alter it as required. Muscles need super-improvement by stretching.

- Ensure climate control. One must manage whatever in terms of temperature might be causing extra muscle discomfort.

- Take a look at hard, easy chairs. The individual should sit in a variety of chairs with different levels of back and bottom cushioning, as well as differing angles and lengths of the seat cushion to find what the most comfortable and suitable texture is.

In order to lessen the impact that a painful and impaired lumbar spine and/or hip(s) has on everyday tasks, ergonomic modifications that require little effort and cost can be made both in local environments and in the home. Here are some considerations when making your environment ergonomically suitable:

9 798885 930525